The Ultimate Air Fryer Veggie Cookbook

Quick And Easy Veggie Recipes

Alan Green

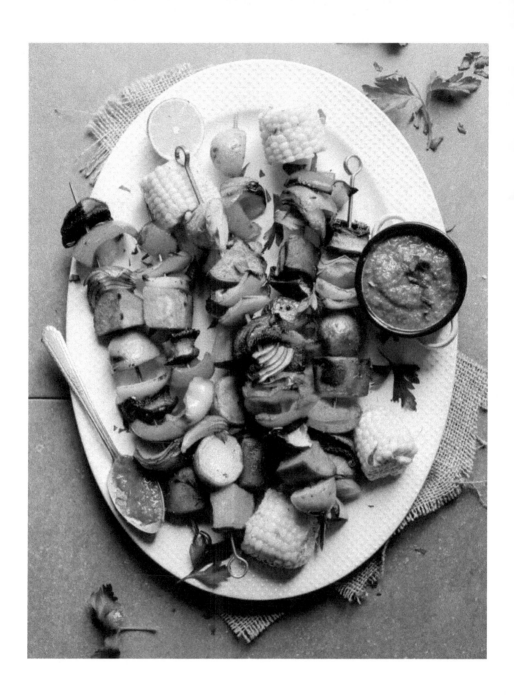

Table of contents

Air-Fryer Roasted Veggies

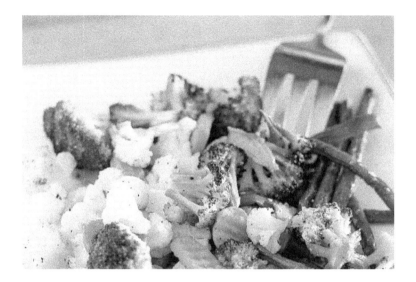

Prep Time: 20 mins

Cook Time: 10 mins

Total Time: 30 mins

Servings: 4

Ingredients

½ cup diced zucchini

½ cup diced summer squash

½ cup diced mushrooms

½ cup diced cauliflower

½ cup diced asparagus

½ cup diced sweet red pepper

2 teaspoons vegetable oil

¼ teaspoon salt

¼ teaspoon ground black pepper

1/4 teaspoon seasoning, or more to taste

Instructions

Preheat the air fryer to 360 degrees F (180 degrees C).

Add vegetables, oil, salt, pepper, and desired seasoning to a bowl. Toss to coat; arrange in the fryer basket.

Cook vegetables for 10 minutes, stirring after 5 minutes.

Nutrition Facts

Calories: 37; Protein; 1.4g; Carbohydrates: 3.4g; Fat: 2.4g; Sodium: 152.2mg.

Marinated Air Fryer Vegetables

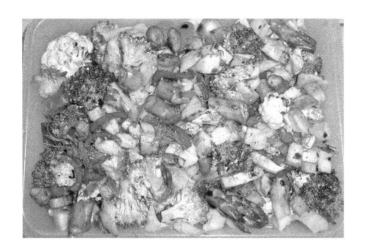

Prep Time: 10 minutes

Cook Time: 15 minutes

Marinading time: 20 minutes

Total Time: 25 minutes

Servings: 4 servings

Ingredients

<u>Vegetables</u>

2 green zucchini cut into ½ inch pieces

1 yellow squash cut into ½ inch pieces

4 oz button mushrooms cut in half

1 red onion cut into ½ inch pieces

1 red bell pepper cut into ½ inch pieces

Marinade

4 Tbsp Olive Oil

2 Tbsp Balsamic Vinegar

1 Tbsp Honey

1 ½ tsp salt

½ tsp dried thyme

½ tsp dried oregano

¼ tsp garlic powder

A few drops of liquid smoke optional

Salt to taste

Instructions

Place marinade ingredients in a large bowl and whisk until combined. Place chopped vegetables in a bowl and stir until all vegetables are fully covered.

Allow vegetables to marinate for 20-30 minutes.

Place marinated vegetables in an air fryer basket and cook at 400 degrees Fahrenheit for 15-18 minutes, stirring every 5 minutes, until tender. Salt to taste.

Nutrition

Calories: 200kcal | Carbohydrates: 16g | Protein: 3g | Fat: 15g | Saturated Fat: 2g | Sodium: 890mg | Potassium: 586mg | Fiber: 3g | Sugar: 12g | Vitamin A: 1225IU | Vitamin C: 67mg | Calcium: 34mg | Iron: 1mg

Air Fryer Vegetables

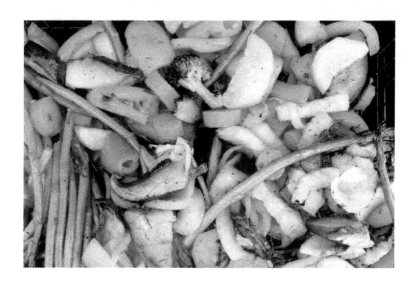

Prep Time: 3 mins

Cook Time: 7 mins

Total Time: 10 mins

Ingredients

1/2 lb broccoli fresh

1/2 lb cauliflower fresh

1 TBSP olive oil

1/4 tsp seasoning can use pepper, salt, garlic salt - I prefer Flavor God Garlic Everything 1/3 c water

Instructions

In a medium bowl, mix vegetables, olive oil, and seasonings.

Pour 1/3 c. water in the Air Fryer base to prevent smoking.

Place vegetables in the air fryer basket.

Cook at 400 degrees for 7-10 minutes.

Shake vegetables to make sure they get evenly cooked about halfway through the 7-10 minutes.

Nutrition

Calories: 65kcal | Carbohydrates: 7g | Protein: 3g | Fat: 4g | Saturated Fat: 1g | Sodium: 37mg | Potassium: 349mg | Fiber: 3g | Sugar: 2g | Vitamin A: 355IU | Vitamin C: 77.9mg | Calcium: 44mg | Iron: 0.8mg

Airfried Vegetables

Prep Time: 10 min

Cook Time: 20 min

Total Time: 30 min

Serves: 4

Ingredients

1 lb / 0.5kg of vegetables (broccoli, brussels sprouts, carrots, cauliflower, parsnips, potatoes, sweet potatoes, zucchini will all work), chopped evenly

1 Tbsp / 30 mL of cooking oil

Some salt and pepper

Instructions

<u>Prep</u>

Preheat air fryer for about 5 minutes at 360F / 182C degrees.

Evenly chop veggies and toss with oil and some salt and pepper. If making potato or sweet potato fries, soak them in water for ~30 minutes to draw out excess starch for crispier results, and then pat dry thoroughly with paper towels before tossing with oil.

<u>Make</u>

Transfer veggies into frying compartment and fry for 15 to 20 minutes, stirring veggies every 5 to 8 minutes or so. Some veggies might need longer and some will need less – just use your judgment when you open the compartment to stir the veggies. You want the outside to be golden and crispy and the inside to be tender.

Enjoy or toss with your favorite dipping sauce when done! If you need sauce ideas, check out 5 of our favorites.

Nutrition Information

Calories: 172, Total Fat: 11g, Saturated Fat: 2g, Unsaturated Fat: 9g, Sodium: 577mg, Carbohydrates: 16g, Fiber: 6g, Sugar: 4g, Protein: 6g

Air Fryer Vegetables

Prep Time: 10 minutes

Cook Time: 15 minutes

Total Time: 25 minutes

Servings: 4

Ingredients

380 g Broccoli

250 g Carrots

1 Large Bell pepper

1 Large Onion

1/2 teaspoon Black pepper

1 tablespoon Olive oil

1 teaspoon Seasoning vegetable, chicken, turkey seasoning, or any of choice.

Salt to taste

Instructions

Wash and cut the vegetables into bite-size.

Cut veggies on a white flat plate.

Add them to a bowl and season with salt, black pepper, or any seasoning of choice, and olive oil. Mix so that the veggies are covered in the seasoning.

Seasoning and olive oil added to the veggies.

Add the seasoned veggies into the air fryer basket and air fry at a temperature of 175c for 15 minutes.

Air fryer roasted vegetables in the air fryer basket.

Toss the veggies in the basket halfway through cooking so that all sides are crisp.

When done, take out the basket and serve.

The finished dish displayed.

Nutrition Information

Calories: 120kcal | Carbohydrates: 19g | Protein: 4g | Fat: 4g | Saturated Fat: 1g | Sodium: 78mg | Potassium: 657mg | Fiber: 6g | Sugar: 8g | Vitamin A: 12338IU | Vitamin C: 144mg | Calcium: 96mg | Iron: 2mg

Roasted Air Fryer Vegetables

Prep Time: 5 minutes

Cook Time: 12 minutes

Total Time: 17 minutes

Servings: 4

Ingredients

1 red bell pepper

1-2 yellow squash

1 zucchini

1/4 medium red onion

1 cup broccoli

1 tbsp olive oil

1/2 teaspoon salt

1/2 teaspoon garlic powder

1/8 teaspoon black pepper

Instructions

Cut up 1 red bell pepper, 2 small yellow zucchini squash, 1 zucchini, 1/2 a medium onion, and 1 cup of broccoli into similar sized chunks.

Add the sliced vegetables into a large bowl and toss them with 1 tablespoon of olive oil, 1/2 teaspoon salt, 1/2 teaspoon garlic powder, and 1/8 teaspoon black pepper.

Once the veggies a coated in the oil and seasoning, place them onto the bottom of your air fryer basket and roast for 10-12 minutes at 400 degrees Fahrenheit.

Nutrition

Calories: 65kcal | Carbohydrates: 7g | Protein: 2g | Fat: 4g | Saturated Fat: 1g | Sodium: 305mg | Potassium: 391mg | Fiber: 2g | Sugar: 4g | Vitamin A: 1269IU | Vitamin C: 75mg | Calcium: 26mg | Iron: 1mg

Air Fryer Roast Vegetables

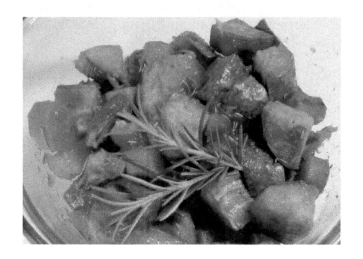

Prep Time: 5 Minutes

Cook Time: 10 Minutes

Total Time: 15 Minutes

Ingredients

1 large sweet potato

1 large potato

1 large carrot

¼ small pumpkin

½ tsp spice or herb mix, optional

Instructions

Wash the vegetables or peel if preferred, and cut into chunks no thicker than 1 inch (they can be as long as you like). Pat vegetables dry.

Place vegetable pieces in an air fryer basket and spray with olive oil. Add spice if desired. Shake and spray with oil again.

Cook in the air fryer at 360°F (180°C) for 5 minutes. Remove the basket and shake.

Return to the air fryer and cook for a further 5-10 minutes until golden brown.

Nutrition Information

Calories: 156| Unsaturated Fat: 0g| Sodium: 69mg| Carbohydrates: 35g| Fiber: 5g| Sugar: 6g| Protein: 4g

Air Fryer Veggies

Prep Time: 5 mins

Cook Time: 20 mins

Total Time: 25 mins

Ingredients

3 cups mixed vegetables, cut into 1-inch pieces (cauliflower, broccoli, squash, carrots, beets, etc)

1 tablespoon olive oil

1/2 teaspoon kosher salt

Preparation

Place the vegetables in a bowl and toss to coat with the oil and salt.

Place the vegetables in the air fryer basket and cook at 375F degrees for 15-20 minutes or until golden and fork-tender.

Nutrition Information

Calories: 172, Total Fat: 11g, Sodium: 234mg, Carbohydrates: 16g, Fiber: 6g, Sugar: 4g, Protein: 6g

Air Fryer "Roasted" Asparagus

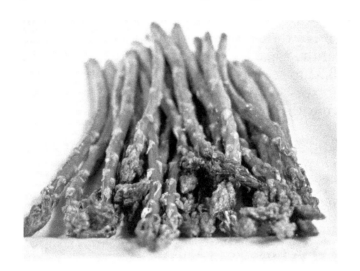

Prep Time: 3 mins

Cook Time: 7 mins

Total Time: 10 mins

Servings: 4 servings

Ingredients

1 pound fresh asparagus, ends trimmed

Oil spray or olive oil

Salt, to taste

Black pepper, to taste

Instructions

Coat the asparagus with oil spray or olive oil and season with salt and pepper. Lay the asparagus evenly in the air fryer basket. Make sure to coat the asparagus tips so they don't burn or dry out too fast. It is best to season before you put it in the air fryer basket. Too much excess salt in the air fryer baskets will often start to break down with coating.

Air Fry at 380°F for 7-10 minutes, depending on thickness, shake, and turn asparagus halfway through cooking.

Taste for seasoning & tenderness, then serve.

Nutritional Value

Calories: 572kcal | Carbohydrates: 1g | Protein: 46g | Fat: 43g | Saturated Fat: 22g | Cholesterol: 168mg | Sodium: 219mg | Potassium: 606mg | Sugar: 1g | Calcium: 16mg | Iron: 4mg

Air Fryer Vegetables

Prep Time: 10 minutes

Cook Time: 10 minutes

Servings: 6

Ingredients

2 zucchini cut into dials

2 yellow squash cut into dials

1 container mushrooms cut in half

1/2 c olive oil

1/2 onion sliced

3/4 tsp Italian seasoning

1/2 tsp garlic salt

1/4 tsp Lawry's seasoned salt

Instructions

Slice zucchini and yellow squash into dials. The thinner they are the softer they will get. I would recommend 3/4" thick so they all are the same consistency when done.

Slice mushrooms in half. Put all vegetables in a bowl and toss together gently. (if you want to add 1/2-1 full precooked sausage link diced into bite-size pcs., add that now too)

Pour olive oil on top and toss gently, then sprinkle in all seasonings in a bowl and gently toss one more time.

Add half of your vegetables into your air fryer, close, and set to 400 degrees for 10 minutes. I did not bother shaking or tossing halfway through and they came out amazing.

Remove, enjoy, and add another half at 400 degrees for 10 minutes to finish the cooking batch.

Nutrition Facts

Fat: 18g, Saturated Fat: 3g1, Sodium: 201mg, Potassium: 355mg, Carbohydrates: 5g, Fiber: 2g, Sugar: 3g, Protein: 2g, Vitamin: A 261IU, Vitamin C: 23mg, Calcium: 26mg, Iron: 1mg

Air Fryer Frozen Broccoli, Carrots, And Cauliflower – (Gluten-Free, Vegan, Keto, And Paleo)

Prep time: 5 min

Cook Time: 10 min

Total Time: 15 min

Serves: 3 people

Ingredients:

3 cups frozen mixed broccoli, carrots, and cauliflower

 1 TBS extra virgin olive oil

1 tsp Italian seasoning blend (or basil, oregano, rosemary, and thyme)

1/2 tsp nutritional yeast (optional)

1/2 tsp sea salt

1/4 tsp freshly cracked pepper

Directions:

Preheat the air fryer to 375°F for 5 minutes.

Place the frozen vegetables in a large mixing bowl. Pour the olive oil over the vegetables and toss to coat. Sprinkle the herbs, salt, pepper, and nutritional yeast over the vegetables and toss again.

Add the vegetables to the crisper plate or basket of the air fryer in an even layer. Cook for 5 minutes. Shake the bucket, or rotate the vegetables. Continue to cook for an additional 4 to 6 minutes until the vegetables are tender and cooked through to a warm temperature. Taste one to test for doneness.

Place the cooked vegetables on a serving platter. You can top with more nutritional yeast before serving.

Nutritional Value

Total fat: 3.7g, Sodium: 1820.8mg, Sugar: 11.3g, Vitamin A: 169.2ug, Carbohydrates: 33.6mg, Protein:18g, Vitamin C: 165.5mg

Healthy Air Fryer Chicken And Veggies

Prep Time: 5 minutes

Cook Time: 15 minutes

Total Time: 20 minutes

Servings: 4 servings

Ingredients

1 pound chicken breast, chopped into bite-size pieces (2-3 medium chicken breasts)

1 cup broccoli florets (fresh or frozen)

1 zucchini chopped

1 cup bell pepper chopped (any colors you like)

1/2 onion chopped

2 cloves garlic minced or crushed

2 tablespoons olive oil

1/2 teaspoon EACH garlic powder, chili powder, salt, pepper 1 tablespoon Italian seasoning (or spice blend of choice)

Instructions

Preheat air fryer to 400F.

Chop the veggies and chicken into small bite-size pieces and transfer to a large mixing bowl.

Add the oil and seasoning to the bowl and toss to combine.

Add the chicken and veggies to the preheated air fryer and cook for 10 minutes, shaking halfway, or until the chicken and veggies are charred and chicken is cooked through. If your air fryer is small, you may have to cook them in 2-3 batches.

Nutrition

Calories: 230kcal | Carbohydrates: 8g | Protein: 26g | Fat: 10g | Saturated Fat: 2g | Cholesterol: 73mg | Sodium: 437mg | Potassium: 734mg | Fiber: 3g | Sugar: 4g | Vitamin A: 1584IU | Vitamin C: 79mg | Calcium: 50mg | Iron: 1mg

Air Fryer Vegetable "Stir-Fry"

Prep Time: 5 minutes

Cook Time: 7 minutes

Total Time: 12 minutes

Ingredients

50 grams extra firm tofu, cut into strips (about 1 cup)

4 stalks asparagus, ends trimmed and cut in half

4 brussels sprouts, halved

3 brown mushrooms, sliced

2 cloves garlic, minced

1 teaspoon italiano seasoning

½ teaspoon sesame oil (or olive oil)

¼ teaspoon soy sauce

Salt and pepper, to taste

Roasted white sesame seeds (for garnish)

Instructions

Combine all ingredients into a large mixing bowl, and toss to combine.

Transfer into air fryer basket and air fry at 350 F for 7-8 minutes, depending on how well done you would like the vegetables. Give the basket a shake halfway through.

Remove from air fryer basket, sprinkle some roasted white sesame seeds on top, and serve with a side of rice.

Nutrient Value

Total fat: 3.7g, sodium: 1820.8mg, sugar: 11.3g, Vitamin A: 169.2ug, Carbohydrates: 33.6mg, Protein:18g, Vitamin C: 165.5mg

Air Fryer Roasted Vegetables

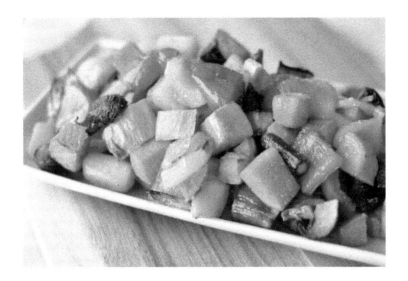

Prep Time: 5 minutes

Cook Time: 20 minutes

Total Time: 25 minutes

Servings: 4

Ingredients

2 tablespoons olive oil

1 medium zucchini sliced

8 oz fresh mushrooms sliced

1 tablespoon minced garlic

Garlic powder to taste

Onion powder to taste

Salt and pepper to taste

Instructions

Preheat air fryer to 390.

Combine all ingredients in a bowl and toss well to coat in oil.

Spread out in a single layer in your air fryer basket (in batches if needed).

Cook for 10 minutes and stir.

Cook for an additional 5 to 10 minutes until vegetables reach your desired texture.

Nutrition

Calories: 84kcal | Carbohydrates: 4g | Protein: 2g | Fat: 7g | Saturated Fat: 1g | Sodium: 6mg | Potassium: 281mg | Fiber: 1g | Sugar: 2g | Vitamin A: 78IU | Vitamin C: 9mg | Calcium: 10mg | Iron: 1mg | Net Carbs: 3g

Air Fryer vegetables

Prep Time: 10 mins

Cook Time: 10 mins

Total Time: 20 mins

Ingredients

2 zucchini

1-2 yellow squash

1/2 sweet onion

1 8 oz container mushrooms

1 bell pepper

1/4 cup olive oil

1 teaspoon Italian seasoning

1/2 teaspoon salt

1/4 teaspoon ground black pepper

Instructions

Cut squash, zucchini, pepper, onion, and mushrooms into bite-sized pieces. Place in a large bowl.

Pour olive oil over vegetables. Sprinkle Italian seasoning, salt, and pepper over vegetables. Toss to coat.

Pour vegetables into an air fryer basket. Spread out for one layer. (You might need to cook in 2 batches.)

Cook at 400 degrees F for 10-12 minutes.

Serve warm.

Nutrition

Calories: 168kcal | Carbohydrates: 10g | Protein: 2g | Fat: 14g | Saturated Fat: 2g | Sodium: 304mg | Potassium: 496mg | Fiber: 3g | Sugar: 7g | Vitamin A: 1225IU | Vitamin C: 66mg | Calcium: 39mg | Iron: 1mg

Air Fryer Garlic Zucchini

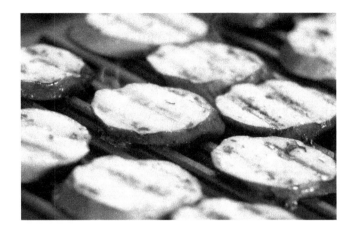

Prep Time: 5 mins

Cook Time: 15 mins

Total Time: 20 mins

Servings: 2 servings

Ingredients

2 zucchini (1 lb. Or 455g total)

Olive oil or cooking spray

1/2 teaspoon garlic powder

Salt, to taste

Black pepper, to taste

Instructions

Trim the ends of the zucchini, if desired. Cut the zucchini into 1/2" thick slices (either into lengthwise slices or into coins). If cutting into lengthwise slices, cut to length to fit the width of your air fryer basket if needed.

Lightly oil or spray the zucchini slices on both sides and then season with garlic powder, salt, and pepper.

Air Fry at 400°F for 8-14 minutes or until browned and cooked through.

Nutrition

Calories: 36kcal | Carbohydrates: 7g | Protein: 2g | Fat: 1g | Saturated Fat: 1g | Sodium: 16mg | Potassium: 512mg | Fiber: 2g | Sugar: 5g | Vitamin A: 390IU | Vitamin C: 35.1mg | Calcium: 31mg | Iron: 0.7mg

Healthy Air Fryer Chicken And Veggies

Prep Time: 5 minutes

Cook Time: 15 minutes

Total Time: 20 minutes

Servings: 4 servings

Ingredients

1 pound chicken breast, chopped into bite-size pieces (2-3 medium chicken breasts)

1 cup broccoli florets (fresh or frozen)

1 zucchini chopped

1 cup bell pepper chopped (any colors you like)

1/2 onion chopped

2 cloves garlic minced or crushed

2 tablespoons olive oil

1/2 teaspoon EACH garlic powder, chili powder, salt, pepper 1 tablespoon Italian seasoning (or spice blend of choice)

Instructions

Preheat air fryer to 400F.

Chop the veggies and chicken into small bite-size pieces and transfer to a large mixing bowl.

Add the oil and seasoning to the bowl and toss to combine.

Add the chicken and veggies to the preheated air fryer and cook for 10 minutes, shaking halfway, or until the chicken and veggies are charred and chicken is cooked through. If your air fryer is small, you may have to cook them in 2-3 batches.

Nutrition

Calories: 230kcal | Carbohydrates: 8g | Protein: 26g | Fat: 10g | Saturated Fat: 2g | Cholesterol: 73mg | Sodium: 437mg | Potassium: 734mg | Fiber: 3g | Sugar: 4g | Vitamin A: 1584IU | Vitamin C: 79mg | Calcium: 50mg | Iron: 1mg

Air Fryer Veggie Tots

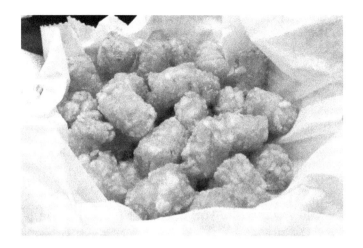

Prep Time: 10 minutes

Cook Time: 12 minutes

Servings: 20 tots

Ingredients

1 cup sweet potato (baked in the oven until soft and skin removed)

1 ½ cups kale

1 egg

½ cup rice crumbs I grab my rice crumbs at Trader Joe's. These are a great gluten-free option. Panko bread crumbs can be substituted.

½ tsp garlic powder

½ tsp paprika

¼ tsp salt

¼ tsp pepper

2 tsp olive oil

Instructions

Spray or drizzle 1/2 tsp olive oil in the air fryer. Place the tots into the air fryer. Do not stack them on top of each other to ensure they become crispy. Spray or drizzle 1 tsp olive oil over the top of the tots and cook at 400 degrees for 10-15 minutes. Repeat if needed (depending on the size of your air fryer.) Pulse kale in a food processor into small flakes.

Air Fryer Veggie Tots

Mash the cooked sweet potato with a fork. If you just cooked the sweet potato, allow it to cool completely. Mix in the kale, egg, and rice crumbs and spices until combined.

Form into "tot-like" shapes with a 1 tbsp scoop or just create small round shapes. They don't have to be perfect!

Spray or drizzle ½ tsp olive oil into the air fryer. Place the tots into the air fryer. Do not stack them on top of each other to ensure they become crispy. Spray or drizzle 1 tsp olive oil over the top of the tots and air fry at 400 degrees for 10-15 minutes. Repeat if needed, depending on the size of your air fryer.

Serve with a dipping sauce! I made an easy 3 ingredient sauce with Wunder Creamery Quark, Primal Kitchen Dairy-Free Mayo, and Primal Kitchen Ketchup. Enjoy!

Nutritional Value

Total fat: 3.7g, Sodium: 1820.8mg, Sugar: 11.3g, Vitamin A: 169.2ug, Carbohydrates: 33.6mg, Protein:18g, Vitamin C: 165.5mg

Air Fryer Vegetables Recipe

Prep Time: 15 Minutes

Cook Time: 20 Minutes

Total Time: 35 Minutes

Ingredients

1 cup broccoli florets

1 cup cauliflower florets

1/2 cup baby carrots

1/2 cup yellow squash, sliced

1/2 cup baby zucchini, sliced

1/2 cup sliced mushrooms

1 onion, sliced

1/4 cup balsamic vinegar

1 tbsp olive oil

 1 tbsp minced garlic

1 tsp sea salt

1 tsp black pepper

1 tsp red pepper flakes

1/4 cup parmesan cheese

Instructions

Pre-heat Air Fryer at 400 for 3 minutes (you can skip this step if you'd like)

In a large bowl, olive oil, balsamic vinegar, garlic, salt and pepper, and red pepper flakes. Whisk together.

Add vegetables and toss to coat.

Add vegetables to the Air Fryer basket. Cook for 8 minutes. Shake vegetables and cook for 6-8 additional minutes.

Add cheese and bake for 1-2 minutes.

Nutrition Information:

Total Fat: 3g|Saturated Fat: 1g|Trans Fat: 0g|Unsaturated Fat: 2g|Cholesterol: 3mg|Sodium: 366mg|Carbohydrates: 8g|Fiber: 2g|Sugar: 3g|Protein: 2g

Asian-Style Air Fryer Green Beans

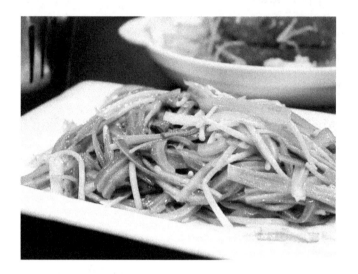

Prep Time: 5 Minutes

Cook Time: 5 Minutes

Total Time: 10 Minutes

Ingredients

1 lb green beans, washed and trimmed

2 teaspoons sesame oil

1 teaspoon garlic salt

Pepper to taste

Instructions

Preheat your air fryer to 400 degrees.

Place the trimmed green beans, sesame oil, garlic salt, and pepper into a bowl and mix to evenly coat green beans.

Put green beans into your preheated air fryer for 5-7 minutes shaking the basket halfway through. You can check the tenderness with a fork to test if the green beans are done. Remove green beans from the air fryer and enjoy!

Nutrition Information

Total Fat: 3g| Unsaturated Fat: 2g| |Sodium: 398mg|Carbohydrates: 10g|Fiber: 4g|Sugar: 4g|Protein: 2g

Air Fryer Broccoli

Prep Time: 5 min

Cook Time: 6 min

Total Time: 11 minutes

Ingredients

12 oz fresh broccoli florets, cut/torn into toughly even, very-small pieces

2 tablespoons extra virgin olive oil

1/4 tsp garlic powder

1/4 tsp onion powder

1/8 tsp kosher salt

1/8 tsp freshly ground black pepper

Instructions

Combine all ingredients in a bowl; toss well to fully incorporate seasonings into the broccoli florets Pour 1 TB water into the bottom of the air fryer pan (this helps prevent contents from smoking.)

Add broccoli mixture evenly into the air fryer basket. Set to 400F for 6 minutes. Once the timer goes off, immediately remove the basket and serve.

Nutritional Value

Calories: 572kcal | Carbohydrates: 1g | Protein: 46g | Fat: 43g | Saturated Fat: 22g | Cholesterol: 168mg | Sodium: 219mg | Potassium: 606mg | Sugar: 1g | Calcium: 16mg | Iron: 4mg

Instant Pot Vortex Air Fryer Vegetables

Prep Time: 5 Minutes

Cook Time: 18 Minutes

Total Time: 23 Minutes

Ingredients

Vegetables Of Choice. Used Here Are:

1 cup broccoli

1 cup cauliflower

1 cup carrots

1 Tablespoon Olive oil or oil of choice

Instructions

Place the vegetables in a bowl and toss with the oil

Add seasoning and toss

Add the vegetable to the Vortex rotisserie basket (or your air fryer basket with other brands)

Air fry on 380 or 18 minutes or until vegetables are roasted with golden brown parts

Carefully remove the basket using the removal tool, serve, and enjoy!

Nutrition Information:

Total Fat: 10g| Saturated Fat: 1g| Trans Fat: 0g| Unsaturated Fat: 8g| Cholesterol: 0mg| Sodium: 68mg| Carbohydrates: 14g| Fiber: 6g| Sugar: 4g| Protein: 3g

"Fried" Tempura Veggies

Hands-On: 15 mins

Total Time: 25 mins

Servings: 4

Ingredients

½ Cup flour

½ teaspoon salt, plus more to taste

½ teaspoon black pepper

2 eggs

2 water

1 cup panko bread crumbs

2 teaspoons vegetable oil

¼ teaspoon seasoning, or more to taste

2 – 3 cups vegetable pieces (whole green beans, sweet pepper rings, zucchini slices, whole asparagus spears, red onion rings, or avocado wedges), cut 1/2 inch thick

Instructions

Mix together flour, 1/4 tsp. salt, and the pepper in a shallow dish. Whisk together eggs and water in another shallow dish. Stir together panko and oil in a third shallow dish. Add the desired Seasoning to either panko and/or flour mixture.

Sprinkle vegetables with remaining 1/4 tsp. salt. Dip in flour mixture, then in egg mixture, and finally in panko mixture to coat.

Preheat air fryer to 400°F and oven to 200°F. Arrange half of the vegetables in a single layer in a fryer basket. Cook until golden brown, about 10 minutes. Sprinkle with additional salt, if desired. Transfer vegetables to the oven to keep warm. Repeat with remaining vegetables. Serve with dipping sauce.

Nutrition Facts

Calories: 179; Total Fat: 5g; Saturated Fat: 1g; Sodium: 375mg; Carbohydrates: 25g; Fiber: 2g; Sugar: 2g; Protein: 7g.

Air Fryer Roasted Potatoes

Prep Time: 5 minutes

Cook Time: 22 minutes

Total Time: 27 minutes

Servings: 4

Ingredients

1.5 pounds potatoes (diced into 1-inch pieces - gold, red, or russets)

1/2 teaspoon garlic powder or granulated garlic

1/2 teaspoon salt or more, to taste

1/4 teaspoon pepper

1/2 teaspoon oregano dried

1/2 teaspoon basil dried

Cooking spray (i am using avocado oil cooking spray)

Instructions

Spray the air fryer cooking basket with the cooking spray.

Add diced potatoes to the basket, and give the potatoes a spray.

Add salt, pepper, garlic powder, oregano, and basil, and toss to combine and evenly coat the potatoes.

Cook at 400 degrees (not preheated) until brown and crispy, about 20 to 24 minutes.

Toss them halfway through with a flipper, and shake the basket once more to ensure even cooking.

Nutrition Facts

Calories: 110, Fat: 1g, Sodium: 308mg, Potassium: 702mg, Carbohydrates: 21g, Fiber: 4g, Protein: 4g, Vitamin C: 19.4mg, Calcium: 51mg, Iron: 5.6mg

Air Fryer Cauliflower & Broccoli Bites

Total Time: 1 hour

SERVES: 6 servings

Ingredients

Cooking spray

1 cup panko bread crumbs

¼ cup grated Parmesan

1 Tbsp. Creole seasoning

2 cups cauliflower florets

2 cups broccoli florets

½ cup whole wheat flour

2 large eggs

1 Tbsp. Fresh parsley, finely chopped, optional

Marinara sauce for serving, optional

Directions

Preheat air fryer to 400°F.

Lightly spray the fryer basket with oil.

In a large bowl, combine panko, Parmesan, and creole seasoning. Set aside.

Place flour in a shallow dish and set aside. In a separate dish, whisk 2 eggs and set aside.

Working in small batches, dip cauliflower and broccoli florets into flour and gently shake off excess.

Dip into egg and then press into breadcrumb mixture.
Place florets in the basket and cook until golden and crispy, about 5-6 minutes. Remove from fryer basket and sprinkle with parsley.

Serve immediately with marinara sauce.

Nutrition

Calories: 130, Total Fat: 3.5g, Cholesterol: 65mg, Sodium: 420mg, Total Carbohydrate: 20g (Dietary Fiber 2g, Sugars 1g, Includes 1g Added Sugar), Protein: 8g, Calcium: 4%, Iron: 10%, Potassium: 6%

Air Fryer Vegetable And Cheese Quesadillas

Servings: 2

Ready In: 18min

Prep Time: 10min

Cook Time: 8min

Ingredients

2 (6 inches) flour tortillas

Cooking spray

1/2 cup shredded cheddar cheese

1/2 red bell pepper, sliced

1/2 zucchini, sliced

Directions

Preheat air fryer to 400°F (200°C).

Spray 1 side of a single tortilla generously with cooking spray and place flat in an air fryer basket. Spread half the Cheddar cheese over tortilla. Top cheese layer with bell pepper and zucchini. Spread remaining Cheddar cheese over top.

Place the second tortilla over fillings and spray the top with cooking spray.

Air fry until cheese is melted and tortillas are crisp, 8 to 9 minutes.

Nutrition Facts

Calories: 291; Fat: 13g; Carbohydrates: 31.5g;Protein: 12g ; Cholesterol: 28g ; Sodium: 421g.

Air Fryer Veggie Fajitas

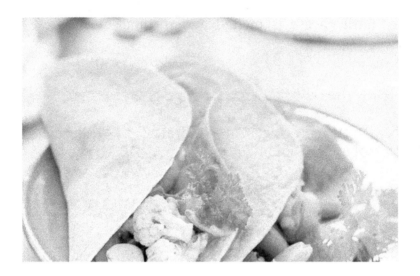

Yield: 2-3 Servings

Prep Time: 10 Minutes

Cook Time: 15 Minutes

Total Time: 25 Minutes

Ingredients

4 portobello mushrooms, sliced into strips

2 sweet peppers (red or yellow), sliced into strips
1 large onion, sliced into strips

Fajita sauce

3 tbsp sweet chili sauce

1 tbsp soy sauce

1 tsp smoked paprika

1/8 tsp chili powder (more if you want it spicy)

1/2 tsp cumin

1/4 tsp ground coriander

To serve

8 tortillas

Toppings of your choice - guacamole, salsa, sour cream or vegan cream, chopped fresh cilantro (coriander)

Instructions

Make the fajita sauce by whisking all ingredients together.

Place the sliced vegetables in a large bowl and coat with the fajita sauce. Allow marinating for a little while in the fridge if you have the time. If you don't, that's OK too - you can go ahead and put them in straight away.

Heat the air fryer to 200C / 390F.

Coat the marinated vegetables with a spray of oil and place them in the fry basket.

Cook for 15 minutes, opening the fryer up to mix the vegetables halfway through.

They're ready when the vegetables are juicy and a little bit charred. You may want to cook for another 5 minutes if they're not yet charred to your liking.

Serve immediately with warmed tortillas and your toppings of choice.

Nutrition Information:

Total Fat: 19g| Saturated Fat: 6g| Trans Fat: 0g| Unsaturated Fat: 11g| Cholesterol: 16mg| Sodium: 1448mg| Carbohydrates: 121g| Fiber: 12g| Sugar: 26g| Protein: 21g

Roasted Winter Vegetables

Servings: 6 Persons

Prep Time: 5 Minutes

Cooking Time: 20 Minutes

Total Time: 25 Minutes

Ingredients

300 g parsnips

300 g celeriac

2 red onions

300 g 'butternut squash'

1 tbsp fresh thyme needles

1 tbsp olive oil

pepper & salt

Directions

Preheat the Airfryer to 200°C.

Peel the parsnips, celeriac, and onions. Cut the parsnips and celeriac into 2 cm cubes and the onions into wedges. Halve the 'butternut squash', remove the seeds and cut into cubes. (There's no need to peel it.)

Mix the cut vegetables with thyme and olive oil. Season to taste.

Place the vegetables into the basket and slide the basket into the Airfryer. Set the timer for 20 minutes and roast the vegetables until the timer rings and the vegetables are nicely brown and done. Stir the vegetables once while roasting.

Nutritional Value

Calories: 572kcal | Carbohydrates: 1g | Protein: 46g | Fat: 43g | Saturated Fat: 22g | Cholesterol: 168mg | Sodium: 219mg | Potassium: 606mg | Sugar: 1g | Calcium: 16mg | Iron: 4mg

Roast Potatoes In A Basket Air Fryer

Prep Time: 5 minutes

Cook Time: 40 minutes

Total Time: 45 minutes

Servings: 4 servings

Ingredients

1.25 kg potato (3 lbs)

1 teaspoon oil

Instructions

Wash potato, peel, cut into large chunks, adding chunks to a large bowl.

Add 1 teaspoon of oil to the bowl of potato chunks and just using your clean hands, toss well until all surfaces are coated. (Tip! first, have the air basket pulled out and beside you, ready to receive the potatoes because your hands will be oily.)

Cook (no need to pre-heat) at 160 C (320 F) for 25 minutes.

Take out the potatoes and tip them back into the bowl you have been using. Toss them in there briefly and gently using a large spoon.

Transfer potato chunks back into fryer basket. Place back into the machine, raise the temperature on the machine to 180 C (350 F), and cook for another 7 minutes.

Take out the potatoes and tip them back into the bowl you have been using. Toss them in there using a large spoon. (At this point, a few might look just about done, but once you toss them you'll see that there are loads that aren't quite as far along.)

Transfer potato chunks back into fryer basket. Leave temperature unchanged. Roast for a final 7 minutes.

Serve piping hot.

Nutrition

Serving: 1g | Calories: 250kcal | Protein: 6.3g | Fat: 1.5g | Sodium: 19mg | Fiber: 6.9g

Crispy Air Fryer Broccoli

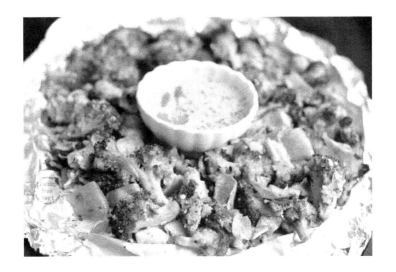

Prep Time: 5 mins

Cook Time: 8 mins

Total Time: 13 mins

Ingredients

4-6 cups broccoli florets

1 tablespoon olive oil

1 tablespoon balsamic vinegar

1/8 teaspoon salt

Instructions

Heat air fryer to 200°C/390°F.

Chop broccoli into equal-sized 1 to 1.5-inch florets and place in a bowl.

Toss broccoli florets with olive oil, balsamic vinegar, and salt.

Add broccoli to the basket. Cook for 7-8 minutes, shaking up the basket every 2-3 minutes. When broccoli florets start to become golden and brown, broccoli is done. Enjoy!

Nutrition

Calories: 65kcal | Carbohydrates: 7g | Protein: 3g | Fat: 4g | Saturated Fat: 1g | Sodium: 104mg | Potassium: 288mg | Fiber: 2g | Sugar: 2g | Vitamin C: 81mg | Calcium: 43mg | Iron: 1mg

Keto Air Fryer Chicken & Veggies

Prep Time: 15 minutes

Cook Time: 15 minutes

Total Time: 30 minutes

Serves: 4

Ingredients

1 lb boneless, skinless chicken breast, cut into bite-sized pieces

2.5 cups broccoli florets

1 medium red bell pepper, chopped

1/2 medium onion, chopped

1 tbsp olive oil

1.5 tsp italian seasoning

1 tsp garlic powder

1/2 tsp paprika

1/2 tsp chili powder

1/2 tsp salt

1/4 tsp black pepper

1/4 tsp onion powder

Direction

Preheat the air fryer to 400 degrees F (if your air fryer allows).

Add chicken breast, broccoli, bell pepper, and onion to a large mixing bowl. Coat with olive oil and seasonings, toss to combine.

Place in air fryer basket and cook for 12-15 minutes, or until chicken is completely cooked through.

Stir halfway through cooking time. Serve hot.

Nutrition

Calories: 189.5, Fat: 4.9g, Carbohydrates: 7.8g, Fiber: 2.7g, Protein: 24.3g, Net Carbs: 5.1g

Veg Cutlet Recipe (Air Fryer Recipe + No Breadcrumbs)

Prep Time: 15 Mins

Cook Time: 40 Mins

Total Time: 55 Mins

Ingredients For Cutlets

2 cups Sweet Potatoes (Boiled, Peeled and Mashed) 1 cup is 250 ml

3/4 cup Carrot (finely grated)

1/2 cup Sweet Corn (steamed)

1/2 cup Capsicum (finely chopped)

1/3 cup Green Peas (Steamed)

1/2 cup Quick Cooking Oats Or Instant Oats

1 tbsp Ginger Paste

1 & 1/2 tbsp Oil For Cooking cutlets (1 tbsp oil is 15 ml)

Salt to taste

2 to 3 tbsp Coriander Leaves (finely chopped)

Spices

1 tsp Kashmiri Red chili powder 1 tsp is 5 ml

1 & 1/2 tsp Garam Masala Powder

1/2 tsp Turmeric Powder

1/4 tsp Chaat Masala Powder

1/2 tsp Amchur Powder or Dry Mango Powder

Instructions

In a wide bowl, add boiled and mashed sweet potatoes, cooked peas, steamed sweet corn, grated carrots, and finely chopped capsicum.

Add all the spices, ginger paste, quick-cooking oats, and salt to taste.

Now add the finely chopped coriander leaves (I have used stems as well).

Mix everything together.

Divide and take an equal portion of the cutlet mixture and shape them into an "oval" shape. Once the cutlets are shaped, preheat the Air Fryer at 200 Degrees C for 5 minutes

Place around 12 cutlets, brush or spray oil and cook them for 15 minutes at 200 Degree C.

Turn them after 8 to 10 minutes of cooking, repeat the process of spraying oil or brushing and air fry them until they are golden brown. Serve with the accompaniment of your choice.

Nutritional Value

Calories: 572kcal | Carbohydrates: 1g | Protein: 46g | Fat: 43g | Saturated Fat: 22g | Cholesterol: 168mg | Sodium: 219mg | Potassium: 606mg | Sugar: 1g | Calcium: 16mg | Iron: 4mg

Air-Fried Crispy Vegetables

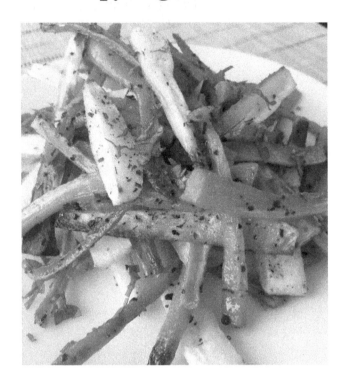

Prep Time: 10 Mins

Cook Time: 15 Mins

Ingredients

2 cups mixed vegetables(bell peppers, cauliflower, mushrooms, zucchini, baby corn)

For batter

1/4 cup cornstarch(cornflour in india)

1/4 cup all-purpose flour/maida

½ tsp garlic powder

½-1 tsp red chilli powder

½-1 tsp black pepper powder

1 tsp salt or as per taste

1 tsp oil

For Sauce Mix

2 tbsp soy sauce

1 tbsp chilli sauce/

1 tbsp tomato ketchup

1 tbsp vinegar(rice/synthetic or apple cider)

1 tsp brown sugar/coconut sugar

Other

1 tbsp sesame oil or any plant-based oil

1 tsp sesame seeds

Spring onion greens for garnish

Instructions

Cut Cauliflower in small florets, cubed bell peppers, cut mushrooms in half, and carrots and zucchini in circles. Do not cut very thin strips.

Make a batter with all-purpose flour, cornstarch(sold as cornflour in India), garlic powder, bell pepper powder, red chili powder, and salt.

Add a tsp of oil and make a smooth lump-free batter. Add and coat all the vegetables nicely in the batter.

Preheat the air fryer at 350F, then add the veggies when indicated. Air fry the veggies, it takes about 10 minutes.

Make the sauce mix. In a heavy-bottomed pan, heat a tbsp of oil, add finely chopped garlic, sauté till it gives aroma, and then add the sauce mix and freshly ground black pepper.

Cook for a minute then add the air fried vegetables and mix well with light hands. Coat all the veggies nicely in sauce.

Sprinkle Sesame Seeds and finely chopped spring onion greens and serve hot.

For Sauce Mix.

Mix all the ingredients together listed under the Sauce section.

For the deep-fried version.

Coat vegetables in batter nicely and then deep fry in hot oil, till light brown in color. Oil should be hot enough so that the veggies remain crispy. Take out and cool down and then add to the sauce mix.

Nutritional Value

Total fat: 3.7g, sodium: 1820.8mg, sugar: 11.3g, Vitamin A: 169.2ug, Carbohydrates: 33.6mg, Protein:18g, Vitamin C: 165.5mg

Air Fryer Roasted Brussels Sprouts

Prep Time: 5 Minutes

Cook Time: 18 Minutes

Total Time: 23 Minutes

Ingredients

1 pound Brussels sprouts

1 ½ tablespoon olive oil

½ teaspoon salt

½ teaspoon black pepper

Instructions

Preheat the air fryer to 390 degrees.

Wash Brussels sprouts and pat dry.

Remove any loose leaves.

If the sprouts are larger cut them in half.

Place Brussels sprouts into a bowl.

Drizzle olive oil over the vegetables.

Stir to make sure the Brussels sprouts are fully coated. Place the Brussels sprouts in the basket.

Season with salt and pepper.

Cook for 15 to 18 minutes or until the Brussels sprouts soften and begin to brown.

Serve immediately.

Nutrition Information

Calories: 172, Total Fat: 11g, Saturated Fat: 2g, Unsaturated Fat: 9g, Sodium: 577mg, Carbohydrates: 16g, Fiber: 6g, Sugar: 4g, Protein: 6g

Air Fryer Roasted Broccoli (Low Carb + Keto)

Yield: 4

Cook Time: 8 Minutes

Total Time: 8 Minutes

Ingredients

5 cups broccoli florets

2 tablespoons butter

2 teaspoons minced garlic

1/3 cup shredded parmesan cheese

Salt and pepper to taste

Lemon slices (optional)

Instructions

Melt the butter and combine with the minced garlic, set aside for later.

Preheat your air fryer according to the manufactures directions at a temperature of 350 degrees.

Add the chopped broccoli florets to the basket of the air fryer and spray very lightly with cooking oil. Roast the broccoli for 8 minutes total. I remove the basket after 4 minutes and shake or toss with tongs to make sure everything is cooking evenly, then cook for 4 more minutes.

At this point, the broccoli should be fork tender at the thickest part of the stem and slightly crispy on the outside.

Remove the broccoli from the basket and toss with the garlic butter, parmesan and add salt and pepper to taste.

Nutrition Information:

Calories: 106| Total Fat: 7.9g| carbohydrates: 5.2g| fiber: 2.1g| protein: 5.3g

Air-Fryer Roasted Veggies

Prep Time: 20 mins

Cook Time: 10 mins

Total Time: 30 mins

Servings: 4

Ingredients

½ cup diced zucchini

½ cup diced summer squash

½ cup diced mushrooms

½ cup diced cauliflower

½ cup diced asparagus

½ cup diced sweet red pepper

2 teaspoons vegetable oil

¼ teaspoon salt

¼ teaspoon ground black pepper

1/4 teaspoon seasoning, or more to taste

Instructions

Preheat the air fryer to 360 degrees F (180 degrees C).

Add vegetables, oil, salt, pepper, and desired seasoning to a bowl. Toss to coat; arrange in the fryer basket.

Cook vegetables for 10 minutes, stirring after 5 minutes.

Nutrition Facts

Calories: 37| Protein: 1.4g| Carbohydrates: 3.4g| Fat: 2.4g| Sodium: 152.2mg.

Buttery Garlic Green Beans

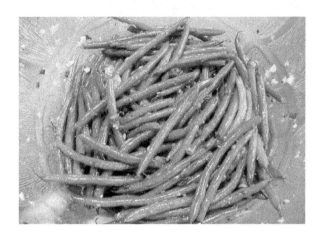

Prep Time: 10 mins

Cook Time: 10 mins

Total Time: 20 mins

Servings: 4

Ingredients

1 pound fresh green beans, trimmed and snapped in half

3 tablespoons butter

3 cloves garlic, minced

2 pinches lemon pepper

Salt to taste

Instructions

Place green beans into a large skillet and cover with water; bring to a boil. Reduce heat to medium-low and simmer until beans start to soften about 5 minutes. Drain water. Add butter to green beans; cook and stir until butter is melted 2 to 3 minutes.

Cook and stir garlic with green beans until garlic is tender and fragrant for 3 to 4 minutes. Season with lemon pepper and salt.

Nutrition Facts

Calories: 116; Protein: 2.3g; Carbohydrates: 8.9g; Fat: 8.8g; Cholesterol: 22.9mg; Sodium: 222.5mg

Superb Sauteed Mushrooms

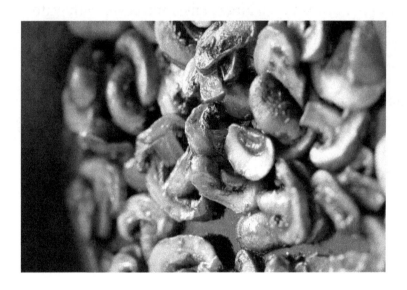

Prep Time: 10 mins

Cook Time: 15 mins

Total Time: 25 mins

Servings: 4

Ingredients

3 tablespoons olive oil

3 tablespoons butter

1 pound button mushrooms, sliced

1 clove garlic, thinly sliced

1 tablespoon red cooking wine

1 tablespoon teriyaki sauce, or more to taste

¼ teaspoon garlic salt, or to taste

Freshly ground black pepper to taste

Instructions

Heat olive oil and butter in a large saucepan over medium heat. Cook and stir mushrooms, garlic, cooking wine, teriyaki sauce, garlic salt, and black pepper in the hot oil and butter until mushrooms are lightly browned, about 5 minutes. Reduce heat to low and simmer until mushrooms are tender, 5 to 8 more minutes.

Nutrition Facts

Calories: 199; Protein: 3.9g; Carbohydrates: 5.3g; Fat: 19.2g; Cholesterol: 22.9mg; Sodium: 375.7mg.

Pan-Fried Asparagus

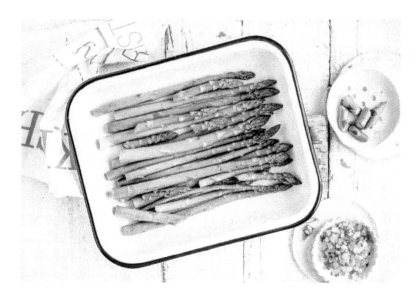

Prep Time: 5 mins

Cook Time: 15 mins

Additional Time: 5 mins

Total Time: 25 mins

Servings: 4

Ingredients

¼ cup butter

2 tablespoons olive oil

1 teaspoon coarse salt

¼ teaspoon ground black pepper

3 cloves garlic, minced

1 pound fresh asparagus spears, trimmed

Instructions

Melt butter in a skillet over medium-high heat. Stir in the olive oil, salt, and pepper. Cook garlic in butter for a minute, but do not brown. Add asparagus, and cook for 10 minutes, turning asparagus to ensure even cooking.

Nutrition Facts

Calories: 188; Protein 2.8g; Carbohydrates 5.2g; Fat 18.4g; Cholesterol 30.5mg; Sodium 524.6mg.

Easy Roasted Broccoli

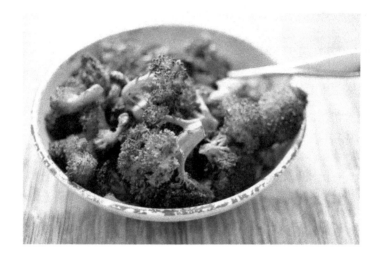

Prep Time: 10 mins

Cook Time: 20 mins

Total Time: 30 mins

Servings: 4

Ingredients

14 ounces broccoli

1 tablespoon olive oil

Salt and ground black pepper to taste

Instructions

Preheat oven to 400 degrees F (200 degrees C).

Cut broccoli florets from the stalk. Peel the stalk and slice into 1/4-inch slices. Mix florets and stem pieces with olive oil in a bowl and transfer to a baking sheet; season with salt and pepper. Roast in the preheated oven until broccoli is tender and lightly browned, about 18 minutes.

Nutrition Facts

Calories: 63| Protein: 2.8g| Carbohydrates: 6.5g| Fat: 3.7g| Sodium: 71.2mg.

Fried Broccoli

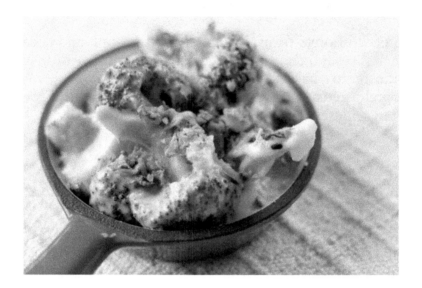

Prep Time: 5 mins

Cook Time: 5 mins

Total Time: 10 mins

Servings: 4

Ingredients

1 (16 ounces) package frozen broccoli, thawed

1 tablespoon olive oil
½ teaspoon crushed red pepper flakes

Salt, to taste

Instructions

Rinse and pat dry the broccoli.

Heat the olive oil in a large skillet over medium heat, add the crushed red pepper, and heat for 1 minute. Cook and stir the broccoli in the skillet until it begins to get crispy, 5 to 7 minutes. Season with salt to serve.

Nutrition Facts

Calories: 61| Protein 3.2g| Carbohydrates: 5.6g| Fat: 3.8g| Sodium: 27.4mg.

Roasted Garlic Lemon Broccoli

Prep Time: 10 mins

Cook Time: 15 mins

Total Time: 25 mins

Servings: 6

Ingredients

2 heads of broccoli, separated into florets

2 teaspoons extra-virgin olive oil

1 teaspoon sea salt

½ teaspoon ground black pepper

1 clove garlic, minced

½ teaspoon lemon juice

Instructions

Preheat the oven to 400 degrees F (200 degrees C).

In a large bowl, toss broccoli florets with extra virgin olive oil, sea salt, pepper, and garlic. Spread the broccoli out in an even layer on a baking sheet.

Bake in the preheated oven until florets are tender enough to pierce the stems with a fork, 15 to 20 minutes. Remove and transfer to a serving platter. Squeeze lemon juice liberally over the broccoli before serving for a refreshing, tangy finish.

Nutrition Facts

Calories:124|Protein:2.9g|Carbohydrates:7g|Fat:1.9g| Sodium: 326.5mg.

Vegetables And Cabbage Stir-Fry With Oyster Sauce

Prep Time: 15 mins

Cook Time: 5 mins

Total Time: 20 mins

Servings: 6

Ingredients

2 tablespoons olive oil

1 pound broccoli florets

1 pound cauliflower florets

½ head cabbage, cut into bite-size pieces

2 cloves garlic, minced

2 tablespoons oyster sauce

Instructions

Heat olive oil in a large skillet or wok over medium-high heat; saute broccoli, cauliflower, cabbage, and garlic in the hot oil until tender-crisp, about 5 minutes.

Remove pan from heat and drizzle oyster sauce over the vegetable mix and toss to coat.

Nutrition Facts

Calories: 111| Protein: 5g| Carbohydrates: 15.2g; Fat: 5g| Sodium: 102.1mg.

Bright And Zesty Broccoli

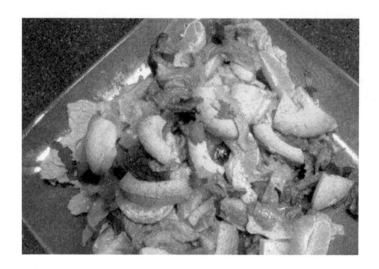

Prep Time: 15 mins

Cook Time: 10 mins

Total Time: 25 mins

Servings: 4

Ingredients

1 tablespoon extra-virgin olive oil

1 ½ tablespoon grated orange zest

½ teaspoon red pepper flakes

1 head broccoli, cut into small pieces with stalks peeled

¼ teaspoon sea salt

¼ teaspoon freshly ground black pepper

2 tablespoons freshly squeezed orange juice

Instructions

Heat the olive oil in a large skillet over medium heat; add the orange zest and red pepper flakes and allow to heat briefly for about 1 minute. Stir the broccoli into the mixture; season with salt and pepper. Continue cooking about 5 minutes more; transfer to a serving bowl. Pour the orange juice over the broccoli and toss to coat. Serve hot.

Nutrition Facts

Calories: 63| Protein: 2.3g| Carbohydrates: 6.6g| Fat: 3.7g| Sodium: 135.1mg.

Spinach & Mushroom Quiche

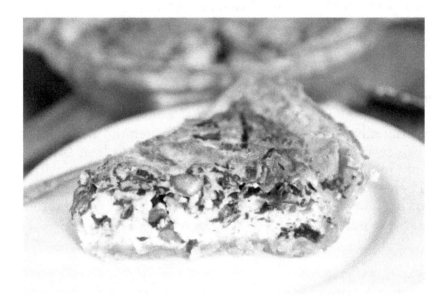

Active Time: 25 mins

Total Time: 1 hr 5 mins

Servings: 6

Ingredients

2 tablespoons extra-virgin olive oil

8 ounces sliced fresh mixed wild mushrooms such as cremini, shiitake, button, and/or oyster mushrooms
1 ½ cups thinly sliced sweet onion

1 tablespoon thinly sliced garlic

5 ounces fresh baby spinach (about 8 cups), coarsely chopped

6 large eggs

¼ cup whole milk

¼ cup half-and-half

1 tablespoon Dijon mustard

1 tablespoon fresh thyme leaves, plus more for garnish

¼ teaspoon salt

¼ teaspoon ground pepper

1 ½ cups shredded Gruyère cheese

Instructions

Preheat oven to 375 degrees F. Coat a 9-inch pie pan with cooking spray; set aside.

Heat oil in a large nonstick skillet over medium-high heat; swirl to coat the pan. Add mushrooms; cook, stirring occasionally until browned and tender, about 8 minutes. Add onion and garlic; cook, stirring often, until softened and tender, about 5 minutes. Add spinach; cook, tossing constantly, until wilted, 1 to 2 minutes. Remove from heat.

Whisk eggs, milk, half-and-half, mustard, thyme, salt, and pepper in a medium bowl. Fold in the mushroom mixture and cheese. Spoon into the prepared pie pan. Bake until set and golden brown, about 30 minutes. Let stand for 10 minutes; slice. Garnish with thyme and serve.

Nutrition Facts

Calories: 227| Protein: 17.1g| Carbohydrates: 6.8g| Dietary Fiber: 1.5g| Sugars: 3.2g| Fat: 20g| Saturated Fat: 8.2g| Vitamin C: 10.8mg| Calcium: 357.8mg| Iron: 2mg| Magnesium: 41.8mg| Potassium: 289.1mg| Sodium: 442.5mg

Cabbage Diet Soup

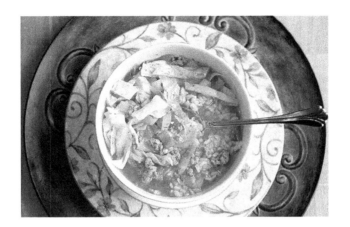

Active Time: 35 mins

Total Time: 55 mins

Servings: 6

Ingredients

2 tablespoons extra-virgin olive oil

1 medium onion, chopped

2 medium carrots, chopped

2 stalks celery, chopped

1 medium red bell pepper, chopped

2 cloves garlic, minced

1 ½ teaspoon Italian seasoning

½ teaspoon ground pepper

¼ teaspoon salt

8 cups low-sodium vegetable broth

1 medium head green cabbage, halved and sliced

1 large tomato, chopped

2 teaspoons white-wine vinegar

Instructions

Heat oil in a large pot over medium heat. Add onion, carrots, and celery. Cook, stirring until the vegetables begin to soften, 6 to 8 minutes. Add bell pepper, garlic, Italian seasoning, pepper, and salt and cook, stirring, for 2 minutes.

Add broth, cabbage, and tomato; increase the heat to medium-high and bring to a boil. Reduce heat to maintain a simmer, partially cover, and cook until all the vegetables are tender, 15 to 20 minutes more. Remove from heat and stir in vinegar.

Nutrition Facts

Calories: 133| Protein: 3g| Carbohydrates: 19.8g| Dietary Fiber: 7g| Sugars: 11g| Fat: 5.2g| Saturated Fat: 0.7g| Vitamin C: 88.2mg| Calcium: 110.7mg| Iron: 1.5mg| Magnesium: 30.2mg| Potassium: 504.1mg|Sodium: 451.1mg

Mexican Cabbage Soup

Total Time: 20 mins

Servings: 8

Ingredients

2 tablespoons extra-virgin olive oil

2 cups chopped onions

1 cup chopped carrot

1 cup chopped celery

1 cup chopped poblano or green bell pepper

4 large cloves garlic, minced

8 cups sliced cabbage

1 tablespoon tomato paste

1 tablespoon minced chipotle chiles in adobo sauce

1 teaspoon ground cumin

½ teaspoon ground coriander

4 cups low-sodium vegetable broth or chicken broth

4 cups water

2 (15 ounces) cans of low-sodium pinto or black beans, rinsed ¾ teaspoon salt

½ cup chopped fresh cilantro, plus more for serving

2 tablespoons lime juice

Instructions

Heat oil in a large soup pot (8-quart or larger) over medium heat. Add onions, carrot, celery, poblano (or bell pepper), and garlic; cook, stirring frequently, until softened, 10 to 12 minutes. Add cabbage; cook, stirring occasionally until slightly softened, about 10 minutes more. Add tomato paste, chipotle, cumin, and coriander; cook, stirring, for 1 minute more.

Add broth, water, beans, and salt. Cover and bring to a boil over high heat. Reduce heat and simmer, partially covered, until the vegetables are tender about 10 minutes. Remove from heat and stir in cilantro and lime juice. Serve garnished with cheese, yogurt, and/or avocado, if desired.

Nutrition Facts

Calories: 167; Protein: 6.5g| Carbohydrates: 27.1g| Dietary Fiber: 8.7g| Sugars: 6.6g| Fat: 3.8g| Saturated Fat: 0.6g| Vitamin A: 2968.9IU| Vitamin C: 47.2mg| Folate: 48.4mcg| Calcium: 115mg| Iron: 2.3mg| Magnesium: 50.5mg| Potassium: 623.7mg| Sodium: 408.1mg|

Everything Bagel Avocado Toast

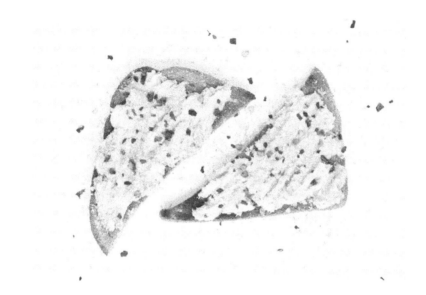

Active Time: 5 mins

Total Time: 5 mins

Servings: 1

Ingredients

¼ medium avocado, mashed

1 slice whole-grain bread, toasted

2 teaspoons everything bagel seasoning

Pinch of flaky sea salt (such as Maldon)

Instructions

Spread avocado on toast. Top with seasoning and salt.

Nutrition Facts

Calories: 172; Protein: 5.4g| Carbohydrates: 17.8g| Dietary Fiber: 5.9g| Sugars: 2.3g| Fat: 9.8g| Saturated Fat: 1.4g| Vitamin C: 5.5mg| Calcium: 60.5mg| Iron: 1.3mg| Magnesium: 41.4mg| Potassium: 341.5mg| Sodium: 251.8mg| Added Sugar: 1g.

Quick Vegetable Saute

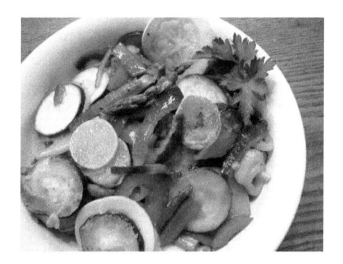

Total Time: 15 mins

Servings: 4

Ingredients

1 tablespoon extra-virgin olive oil

1 small shallot, minced

4 cups mixed frozen vegetables, such as corn, carrots, and green beans

½ teaspoon dried dill or tarragon

¼ teaspoon salt

¼ teaspoon freshly ground pepper

Instructions

Heat oil in a large skillet over medium heat. Add shallot and cook, stirring, until softened, about 1 minute. Stir in frozen vegetables. Cover and cook, stirring occasionally, until the vegetables are tender, 4 to 6 minutes. Stir in dill (or tarragon), salt, and pepper.

Nutrition Facts

Calories: 107; Protein: 2.6g| Carbohydrates: 16.8g| Dietary Fiber: 3.5g|Sugars: 4.2g| Fat: 4.2g| Saturated Fat: 0.6g| Vitamin A: 6423.6IU| Vitamin C: 9.6mg| Folate: 28.3mcg| Calcium: 38.8mg| Iron: 0.9mg| Magnesium: 24mg| Potassium: 293.9mg| Sodium: 177.7mg| Thiamin: 0.1mg.

Lightning Source UK Ltd.
Milton Keynes UK
UKHW020214080521
383350UK00003B/294